UNDISCOVERED DIVA
PRESENTS

RECLAIM YOUR NATURAL BEAUTY

TERRIE LAUREN
FORWARD BY ASH CASH

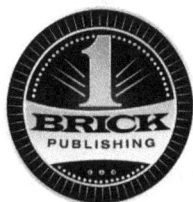

1 BRICK PUBLISHING

Published by 1Brick Publishing
A Division of Ash Cash Enterprises, LLC
P.O. Box 2717 • New York, NY 10027

First Printing: November 2012
Published by:
1Brick Publishing A division of
Ash Cash Enterprises, LLC
P.O. 2717
New York, NY 10027-2717
(877)853-0493

Email: Info@1BrickPublishing.com
Website: www.1BrickPublishing.com

Library of Congress Cataloging-in-Publication Data

Lauren, Terrie 1981-
     Undiscovered Diva Presents Reclaim Your Natural Beauty by Terrie Lauren
     p.   cm.
     ISBN 978-061570394-7 paperback edition

Library of Congress Control Number:
          1.   Success   I. Title   II. Lauren, Terrie
          2.   Self-Help/Self-Improvement
          3.   Beauty

Printed in the United States of America

This book is dedicated to all of the ladies who ever wrapped a towel around their head pretending it was hair.

Table of Contents

ACKNOWLEDGMENTS

Undiscovered Diva Presents: Reclaim Your Natural Beauty was inspired by my daughter. Who knew a three year old could have so much influence but it was her existence that initiated and developed the self discovery within me. Her free spirit and untainted view on life has made me realize how important it is to love and accept yourself the way you were made and that the reality is no one is physically flawed! The gaps in your teeth, the color of your skin, the moles and freckles are all strategically placed right where they should be and I hope that every woman young and old is able to receive that message through the knowledge provided in this book.

To my husband, my rock and biggest supporter all I can say is thank you! This book would not exist today if it were not for the seeds you planted and the admiration I have gained through watching your journey and successes. You have been a mentor and friend and I truly appreciate you flaws and all. ☺

To my cousins the three beautiful young ladies that inspire me daily to keep going thank you! You really do not know how much influence you have on every choice I make in my life.

Last but certainly not least to my mom thank you for instilling independence, hard work and teaching me to always have an open mind and to never be judgmental because there is a lesson to be learned even in things you may not understand.

FORWARD

In 2009 Chris Rock released a documentary titled "Good Hair" that questions what having good hair is as defined by African Americans, mostly Black women. He visits hair conventions, barber shops, salons, and even goes to India, the weave producing capitol of the world, to get to the bottom of this billion dollar business that black people own less than 2% of. As the movie progresses, it teaches viewers about sodium hydroxide, a chemical compound used to relax hair and shows how much damage it can really cause. I cringed as I watched how distorted ideas of beauty and use of relaxers caused physical and emotional damage to children as young as 3 years-old. The only thing I can do is applaud Chris for shedding light on the dangers of mis-education and beginning a movement that allows men and women to reevaluate the ideals of beauty they may be passing on to their daughters. As a father of a beautiful young African American girl, it disturbed me to see what black women go through with their hair in order to appeal to what society deems as beautiful. They say beauty is in the eye of the beholder by how can we trust an eye that has been manipulated and forced to see beauty one way? This is exactly why books like this one, are necessary in order to dispel the myths about hair and create a true sense of what beauty is.

Undiscovered Diva presents: Reclaim Your Natural Beauty isn't a book about how going natural is the best way to go, nor is it a book that is anti-relaxer.... Reclaim Your Natural Beauty is a book necessary for ALL women who are ready to take proper care of their hair so that the nature of their true beauty can really shine in. Beauty is indeed in the eye of the beholder.... Let's begin the journey to get back our 20/20.

-Ash'Cash

INTRODUCTION

For years African American women have gone to great lengths to achieve publicized ideals of beauty. I've witnessed on numerous occasions how women have destroyed their God given crowns to emulate the look of so called "good hair" whether chemicals are used to change the texture, braids to aid in growth or weaves to have the appearance of long flowing hair.

Now don't get me wrong, granted I wear my hair natural, but I am NOT against relaxers, texturizers, weaves or braids. However, I am against the lack of education on how to properly nurture your hair while wearing these styles and destroying ones beauty in the process. As a stylist I have a natural love for all hair types, textures and styles (well not all styles some we can really do without lol) but for the most part I love hair! Being able to work with women of all ethnic backgrounds and constantly learn new ways to tame their manes whether curly, straight, fine and wispy, or thick and coarse is what fuels my passion for this industry.

On the flip side, it pains me to see a woman damaged by years of trauma and mismanagement of their hair all for the sake of beauty. Based on my experiences, I noticed this was a constant trend among women of color.

This trend ultimately results in a lack of self esteem that's passed on to our sisters, daughters, cousins and nieces creating a cycle of women who have no confidence about their outward appearance.

While doing research for this book I came across an article about Traction Alopecia a common disorder caused by wearing tight styles (details in Section III) and was astonished to read that a 19 year old girl was diagnosed with this disorder. Her case was so severe that her only option was to get hair grafted in the balding areas! There weren't many details about her specific case but one can assume that she either had her hair relaxed at a very young age or was a victim of wearing tightly braided hair styles over a long period of time. Its stories like these that made me realize this was an issue that needed to be addressed and encouraged me to write this book to provide a simple guide to healthy hair care.

I personally had a client that came to see me for a wash and blow dry on a weave she had installed about a month prior. As we went through our consultation, I noticed that she also suffered from traction alopecia; her hair was very dry and thin and the tension from the sewn in weave had completely ripped hair from her edges. Despite the damage that had been caused and with tracks of hair weave hanging from strands; she was begging me to just sew the dangling hair anywhere it would hold with no regard to the hair trauma she would suffer later.

She was not the only one! I have had many clients since, both young and old who were emotionally and psychologically damaged from the overuse of chemicals or hair enhancements; not knowing what to do or where to turn, but willing to shell out hundreds to make it right and to look and feel good about themselves. It is a fact that when we look good we feel good but we do not have to destroy the essence of our natural beauty in order to get to that state of being.

If you have picked up this book you have decided to stop the abuse and get educated on how to really take care of your hair. Whether your goal is to gain length or just improve the health of your hair, you will need a regimen. A hair care regimen is a routine on how you plan to take care of your hair. It includes important aspects like deep conditioning, protein treatments and chemical touch ups (if applicable). The regimen you choose should be easily incorporated into your lifestyle to address you hairs needs but not so overwhelming that you become discouraged. With that said I give you *Undiscovered Diva - Reclaim your Natural Beauty* – A Quick and Easy Guide to Healthy Hair Care.

In the following pages you will find a simple guide on how to care for your hair whether it's natural, relaxed, color treated or enhanced with extensions (weaves, braids, wigs, etc) and be able to create a simple regimen to put you on track to obtaining healthy hair. You can choose to simply read the designated area that interests you without skipping a beat or read the book in its entirety and gain knowledge on how to care for any hair type.

Let's get started!

- SECTION I -
THE BASICS

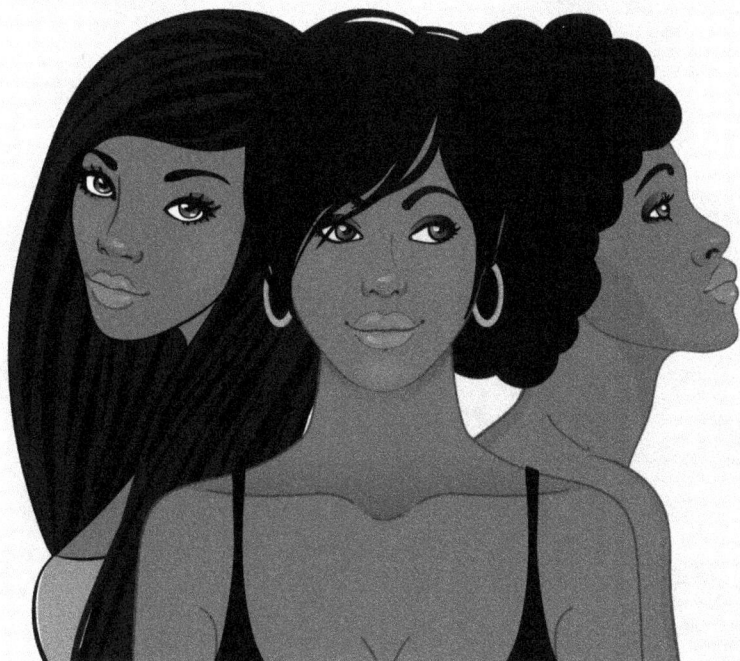

What is Hair?

Hair is composed of Keratin, a special protein that also produces our fingernails and toenails and forms the protective outer layer of our skin. Each strand of hair consists of three concentric layers, **the cuticle, the cortex and the medulla.** The hair cuticle is the outermost part of the hair shaft. It is a hard shingle-like layer of overlapping cells, some five to twelve deep. It is formed from dead cells which form scales that give the hair shaft strength and do the best job of providing protection for the hair strand. The hair cuticle is the first line of defense against all forms of damage; it acts as a protective barrier for the softer inner structure including the medulla and cortex. The cuticle is responsible for much of the mechanical strength of the hair fiber. A healthy cuticle is more than just a protective layer, as the cuticle also represents the structure that controls the water content of the fiber. Much of the shine that makes healthy hair so attractive is due to the cuticle.

Cuticles are often damaged by excessive mechanical manipulation such as brushing, using heat (like using curling irons) or chemical processing (like perms or texturizers). Everyday elements, such as the sun or wind can also cause wear and tear on your hair and damage the hair cuticles as well. Although the cuticle is the outermost layer of the hair, it does not give the hair its color because it has no melanin (pigment), which is what is responsible for an individual's hair; the color of a person's hair depends on what type of melanin they have which is found in the cortex. There are two kinds of melanin, eumelanin which creates brown or black hair, and pheomelanin which makes hair appear red. Gray hair is a result of a lack of melanin which is often caused by age but can also be caused by stress and illness. The innermost layer of hair is called the medulla and reflects light giving hair the various color tones it has. That's why hair color looks a lot different in sunlight than it does in the shade.

The cortex which is the middle layer of the hair is made up of polypeptide chains. These polypeptide chains are cross linked together, like a ladder by three different types of side bonds: **hydrogen bonds, salt bonds and disulfide bonds**. These side bonds hold the hair fibers in place and are responsible for the strength and elasticity of human hair.

A hydrogen bond is a physical bond that is easily broken by water or heat. Although individual hydrogen bonds are very weak, there are so many of them that they account for about one third of the hair's overall strength.

A salt bond is also a physical bond, but it is broken by changes in pH. Salt bonds are easily broken by strong alkaline or acidic solutions and also account for one third of the hairs strength.

A disulfide bond is a chemical side bond. Although there are far fewer disulfide bonds than hydrogen or salt bonds, disulfide bonds are much stronger and **cannot** be broken by heat or water (please keep this in mind when reading the definition of natural hair). Permanent waves (curly perms/jheri curls), texturizers and chemical relaxers are the only elements that change the shape of the hair by chemically changing the hairs disulfide bonds.

The medulla is the innermost layer of the hair follicle. It is composed of round cells and it's quite common for very fine and naturally blonde hair to entirely lack a medulla. Generally only thick, coarse hair contains a medulla however as far as cosmetology is concerned the medulla is an "empty space" and does not play a factor in treatments or services.

HAIR GROWTH RATE/CYCLE

The internet is filled with advice and products designed to make hair grow faster. But the reality is that human hair has a specific rate of growth that does not vary growing at a rate of ¼ to ½ inch each month. Factors that determine how fast an individual's hair grows include genetics, gender and hormones.

While hair care and factors such as split ends can make hair seem to grow at a slower rate, remember **actual hair growth from the root does not vary.** It will continue to grow ¼ - ½ inch each month, it's how you take care of the older hair that makes the difference. Each individual hair follicle cycles through periods of growth and rest known as anagen, catagen and telogen.

Anagen - This is the growth phase that lasts between two and eight years. During the anagen phase the growth cells in the papilla rapidly divide and produce the hair shaft which becomes keratinized as it pushes up and out of the follicle into the pore. At the same time, the follicle grows down into the deeper levels of the dermis (skin) to get nourishment. People who have long anagen growth rates are able to grow very long hair and others have short growth phases and cannot grow very long hair. Hair grows at a rate of about a ½ inch per month, so a hair left uncut will grow to a length of between 12 inches and 48 inches.

Catagen - The Anagen phase is followed by a brief two to four week Catagen phase or transitional phase. This is part of a renewal process where the follicle is literally degraded and the hair stops growing but does not fall out. During the Catagen phase the hair follicle shrinks to about 1/6 of the normal length. The lower part is destroyed, the dermal papilla breaks away, the bulb detaches from the blood supply and the hair shaft eventually is pushed up as the follicle disintegrates.

Telogen - The follicle then goes into the Telogen or resting phase for two to four months, during this time the hair still does not grow but remains attached to the follicle while the dermal papilla is in a resting phase below. Approximately 10-15 percent of all hairs are in this phase at any one time.

After the Telogen phase the cycle is complete and the hair goes back into the Anagen phase. It is at this time when the new hair shaft is forming that the old hair is pushed out and lost.

On average 50-100 hairs are lost due to this natural growth process every day. This is normal hair loss and accounts for the hair loss seen every day in the shower and with hair combing. In healthy follicles these hairs will soon be replaced by new hair.

A variety of factors can alter the normal hair growth cycle and cause temporary or permanent hair loss including medication, radiation, chemotherapy, exposure to chemicals, hormonal and nutritional factors, thyroid disease, generalized or local skin disease, and stress.

When it comes to hair growth you will hear many things and be offered many ways to assist in increasing the speed or "stimulating" hair growth. Most of the time these are marketing ploys and fancy ways to make you buy a product or add on service; below is the truth to some common hair growth myths you may have heard:

Myth – shaving, clipping and cutting the hair makes it grow back faster, darker and coarser.

Fact – Shaving or cutting the hair has no effect on hair growth. When hair is bluntly cut to the same length it grows back evenly. Although that may make it seem to grow back faster and coarser cutting the hair has no effect on hair growth.

Myth – Scalp massage increases hair growth.

Fact – There is no evidence that any type of stimulation or scalp massage increases hair growth. Minoxidil and finasteride are the only treatments that have been proven to increase hair growth and are approved by the FDA.

Myth – Gray hair is coarser and more resistant than pigmented hair.

Fact – Other than the lack of pigmentation, gray hair is exactly the same as pigmented hair. Although gray hair may be resistant it is not resistant simply because it's gray and it is not more resistant than the pigmented hair on the same persons head.

Myth – The amount of natural curl is determined by racial background.

Fact – Anyone of any race or mixed race can have from straight to extremely curly hair. It is also true that within races, individuals have hair with different degrees of curliness.

Healthy Body Healthy Hair

As the subtitle suggests you really cannot have one without the other. I initially planned to dive in and just give you a basic guide for healthy hair care but after much consideration I felt I would be doing my readers a disservice. The fact of the matter is this; what you put in your body is what you will get out. A well-balanced diet that includes plenty of growth-promoting protein and iron can make a huge difference in the health of your hair. It would be easy for me to give you my personal hair care regimen in detail and list every single product that I use however that list would not include that instead of consuming fried foods and fast food which was a major part of my diet in the past, I now eat one balanced meal a day and as a supplement for the other two meals I drink plenty of water, smoothies made with fresh fruits, and juice raw vegetables giving me the vitamins I need naturally. Adapting these new eating habits play a major role in the overall health of my hair. (Note: I stress that these changes play a role only in the HEALTH of my hair it continues to grow at its normal rate as stated above but I do not experience any excessive breakage.) If you eat a healthy diet; you will grow stronger and healthier cells throughout your entire body inside and out and as a result see amazing results in your hair, skin and nails.

One meal a day and raw fruit and vegetable juice may be a little extreme for some and hey I'm no nutritionist but I do suggest that you make a conscious effort to make better and more nutritious food choices. Before making any drastic changes in your diet please consult with your physician or nutritionist however below are some basic steps you can take to get started:

1. Drink Water - you will notice throughout this book that I mention hydrating and moisturizing often and the best way to do that is with water. Drink the recommended 8 glasses of water a day. Add crystal light for flavor if you aren't the biggest fan of water. Not only are you doing what's good for your body you will also notice the difference in your hair!

* Tip - *Drinking a glass of water before bed helps you relax and leaves you feeling rejuvenated in the morning. While you sleep, water has the time to reach every part of your body and replenish it fully. You will be able to sleep more soundly and consistently by drinking water before bed, leaving your muscles, vitamins and minerals in harmony.*

2. Take a Multivitamin – In today's society of fast and convenient foods the average person does not receive the necessary amount of vitamins and nutrients through their regular diet. It is recommended to take a daily supplement which does wonders for the body and aids in healthy hair and nail growth. Beware of dietary supplements often marketed to thicken hair or make it grow faster, they may backfire! Although rare there have been instances where excess supplementation of vitamins has been linked to hair loss. Vitamins specifically marketed for hair and nail growth may contain higher levels of biotin which is a B complex vitamin that aids in hair growth however a daily vitamin contains the necessary dosage of B complex vitamins needed. Even though you can find beauty supplements on the shelves of most pharmacies, try to get the nutrients you need from foods whenever possible.

3. Eating Habits – I cannot stress enough that what you put in your body has a direct correlation to what you will get on the outside. Try adding more color to your plate with vegetables and fruits. Opt for the baked or grilled versions of your meat choices. Even when you feel you may not have the time and must do fast foods make better choices; many of these places have salads or overall healthier options on the menu.

4. Exercise - Regular cardiovascular and aerobic exercise can promote hair growth. When you are stressed, it's possible for your hair to thin or fall out this is because your body produces more cortisone. This hormone causes hair follicles to stop growing, which can result in thinning of the hair. Exercise can reduce the levels of the cortisone hormone which will help hair grow faster and fuller.

If you follow this healthy guide, add in a hefty dose of daily exercise to keep that blood pumping, invest in a juicer ;-) then add proper hair care on the surface I guarantee you will see a major difference in your hair.

NOTES

_____
_____
_____
_____
_____
_____
_____
_____
_____
_____
_____
_____
_____
_____
_____
_____
_____
_____
_____
_____
_____
_____
_____
_____
_____

- SECTION II -
NATURAL HAIR

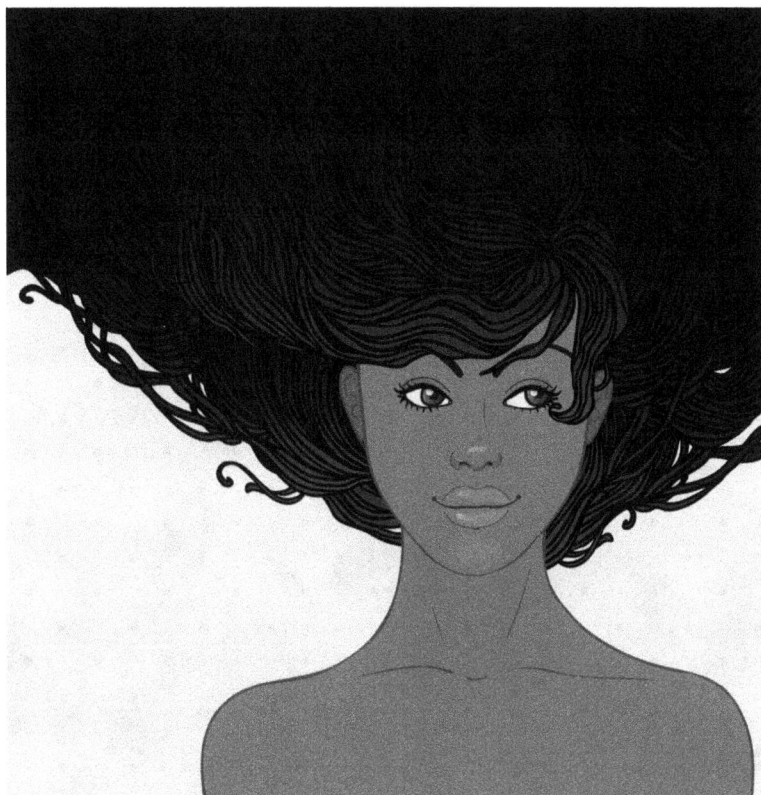

Natural Hair Defined

What is natural hair? Natural hair is often defined as hair that has not been chemically processed or color treated. However for the purpose of this book and to avoid confusion I believe it's important that we make a clear distinction between "natural hair" and "virgin hair".

Natural hair is hair that has not been chemically altered by relaxers, soft curl perms or texturizers to permanently change its texture and curl pattern. On the other hand, **virgin hair** is hair that has never undergone any of the aforementioned chemical procedures or color services including highlighting, permanent and temporary color. Many people in the natural hair community frown on highlighting or adding permanent or semi permanent dyes to the hair claiming that the bleach and peroxide alters the texture. However as long as you are not using a product that is strong enough to break the disulfide bond the texture of your hair has not been altered and there is not a hair color product that has the power to break that bond. With an understanding that "virgin" hair has never been processed in any form, natural hair wearers can enjoy the variety of changing their color and still be considered natural.

Natural Hair Care

There are thousands of websites, blogs and YouTube channels out there in the cyber world that address how to maintain, style and care for your natural hair. As a natural hair wearer I've utilized many of these websites and vlogger channels for information. While it is a great source for styles and hair education it got to the point that I began to feel overwhelmed by the information and ended up more confused about maintenance and products than when I started! (This also encouraged me to write a basic guide on hair care to address all of the hair needs without overwhelming the reader and making one feels as if it's a science project to properly care for your hair.) However, there are simple and basic procedures that everyone can follow for healthy hair; everything in between is based on personal preference especially when it comes to products.

Sometimes in an effort to care for your hair women become "product junkies" trying everything you can get your hands on to make your hair healthy. I've been down that road and spent tons of money making the beauty supplier rich buying things just for the sake of buying them. The one thing that we as consumers must realize whether natural or chemically processed is that what's good for the goose is not always good for the gander. Not everyone has the same texture, density, and curl pattern therefore one product will not give the same results on all heads of hair which leads me to the first rule of having healthy natural hair and that is keeping it moisturized.

There are tons of moisturizers on the market but the best moisturizer for anyone who has curly – coarse hair is water. Not only should you drink the proper amounts of water but it is very important to physically moisturize your hair simply with water. One of the biggest issues most natural hair wearers combat with is hair dryness and they are constantly on the hunt for a miracle product. Sorry to burst your bubble but there is no product out there that will moisturize your hair better than plain old water. For years we have been told to stay away from water because we did not want to mess up our do's or we bought into the age old myth that water dries your hair out. The truth is water is nature's natural moisturizer and it's the shampoos we use that are the culprits of causing dry hair. Below is a list of recommended practices to aid in eliminating dry hair and retaining moisture:

Hydration - Drink at least 8 glasses of water a day. I can't stress how important it is to hydrate your body not only is it good for your overall health but it also aids in having health hair.

Frequency – Increasing how often you wash/co-wash (explained below) your hair is also a very important factor in maintaining moisture. If possible I recommend co washing every three days. I know that sounds like a lot to take your hair out and co wash and restyle but this can also be done while your hair is in its desired style. I personally co wash my hair every 3 days whether it's loose, two strand twisted or even when it's in a funky updo! If every three days still seem to be unrealistic once a week is the minimum. Any duration longer than once a week is really not healthy for your hair especially in its natural state. Because our hair has a curly/coily pattern it takes longer for the sebum (which are the hairs natural oils) to travel down the shaft and provide the needed moisture. When we wet our hair the hydrogen bond is broken and allows water to penetrate the unreached areas and make the hair soft and supple. Water also assists in making natural hair easier to be styled.

Quick Tip – natural hair should **NEVER** be combed dry! If you are styling your hair or your childs hair whether tangled or not always lightly mist with a water based product, water alone or a mixture of your own in a spray bottle.

Co – Wash – Co washing is the process of completely eliminating shampoo from your hair care regimen. Co washing simply means to cleanse your hair with conditioner. Conditioners have the same cleansing power as shampoos without the sulfates. If you are on the fence about just using conditioner as a cleanser try shampooing once a month and co-washing every other time in between doing this process will assist in retaining moisture in the hair.

Shampoo - decrease the number of times you shampoo when you wash your hair, we tend to want to wash our hair three or four times to get that squeaky clean feel however that causes more harm than good. The sulfates and parabens found in shampoos strip your hair of its natural oils causing it to become dry and brittle. One lather usually does the trick but if you feel like you have lots of product buildup you should not exceed more than 2 shampoos. Technically shampoo should be used to cleanse the scalp cleaning away any debris and product buildup to allow the follicle to successfully grow out of the scalp. A good rule of thumb is to remember to shampoo the scalp massaging it with the pads of your fingers and condition the hair. The best practice for cleansing would be to gently squeeze the shampoo suds down the strands to cleanse the hair instead of scrubbing your hair like its laundry. When conditioning apply the conditioner to the ends of your hair where it's needed most, specifically heavy cream deep conditioners. When conditioners are used on the scalp they tend to make your final style flat and without volume and body.

Deep Conditioning – Deep conditioning once a week is **VERY** important. You can use the deep conditioner of your choice but please do not skip this step because when you do it shows! A deep conditioner is any type of conditioner left on the hair for 20-30 minutes. For the deep conditioner to be truly effective, it is important that heat is used along with it. Heat allows the hair shaft to swell and the cuticles to open and allow the conditioner inside. By promoting elasticity, deep conditioning improves the strength of the hair making it more resilient which helps in length retention in the long term.

All hair types can benefit from deep conditioning but for black hair, this is an absolute must! As the hair is dry by nature, deep conditioning restores the moisture balance in the hair which stops breakage.

Sealing in Moisture– Generally natural hair should be moisturized daily and this can only be done with water. To help retain that moisture sealing with oil is imperative. If for any reason you choose to skip any of the above steps at least commit to buying a water bottle, add a few squirts of conditioner, fill it with water and spray your hair once in the morning and once at night. After each spritz apply an oil or hair butter to seal in the moisture. Remember despite popular belief oils and butters **cannot** moisturize your hair. They provide great shine but they do not penetrate the shaft to moisturize. Oils and products like Shea butter sit on top of the shaft acting as a sealant and are very good at holding moisture (water) in the hair.

RETAINING LENGTH

Length retention is another goal that many natural and relaxed hair wearers would like to achieve. I've had many clients complain about how their hair just won't grow but let me be the first to say that is not true. Unless you suffer from some sort of diagnosed scalp disorder or disease your hair does grow at a rate of a ¼ - ½ inch per month however you may encounter breakage and split ends as a result of not wearing protective styles and taking proper care of your hair. For those ladies out there who desire to have long hair the best way to achieve any length is to moisturize, moisturize, moisturize! Follow step 4 which is to increase your co washing frequency or keep your hair in contact with water as often as reasonably possible. I know this is out of the norm for lots of us but after speaking to several women of a variety of racial and ethnic backgrounds that have really long hair the one consistent trait they all share is that they wet their hair every morning! This gives the hair the needed moisture and helps the oldest parts of your hair (the ends) from being brittle and breaking off.

A friend of mine who is Asian and Native American told me she doesn't do much to her hair but wet it in the shower, throw in some conditioner and put it in a bun; which leads me to the second thing that helps retain length and get you closer to your hair goal and that's protective styling.

Protective Styling is the art of making sure the ends of your hair which are the oldest and most fragile is not exposed to the weather elements and rubbing against your sweaters, shirts and pillow cases. Some styles to consider are two strand twists, updos, buns, chignons and braids are great alternatives to wearing your hair out. Wigs, half wigs and weaves are also an option but I will discuss those in more detail in Section III. Following these two simple steps and also investing in satin pillowcases, hair bonnets and scarves will ensure that you do not damage the oldest part of your hair and help you reach the bra strap or waist length goals that many women set.

Products Recommendations

You may have noticed that I do not list any specific products because I strongly believe that there is no one set of products that work for every head of hair. I also do not believe that there is any special product that can work miracles or address your specific hair need however as a natural hair wearer I will recommend a list of products that my hair loves and what it specifically does.

- Water – used DAILY to moisturize.
- Shea Moisture or Jane Carter Shampoo – Both Shampoo lines smell great and do not contain any sulfates and parabens.

- Suave Tropical Coconut Conditioner – I use this for daily co washes. I know you may be thinking this is sooo cheap but it really makes my hair super soft and manageable. I also use this as my conditioner for my daily spritzer by adding it in a spray bottle with some water.

- Shea Moisture organic Shea butter deep treatment masque – used for weekly deep conditioning. (I switch up on my deep conditioners every month however Shea Moisture is one of my favorites)

- Vatika Coconut Oil – oil used daily for sealing in moisture.

- Extra Virgin Olive Oil and Jasmine oil – I normally mix these two oils in with my deep conditioner and sit under a dryer with a plastic cap for about 20 min.

- Shea butter – mostly used during the winter for sealing in moisture.

That concludes my very short and frugal hair care list; again these products work for my hair I suggest you try different things to see what works for you but water should be your #1 staple. I also like everything in the Jane Carter Solutions line. I use her products mainly for styling along with Kinky Curly Custard and Eco Styler Olive Oil Gel. If you would like more detailed styling tips and how I utilize each product check out my website www.undiscovereddiva.com in the tips and gratuities section. Please note that these tips and steps can be applied to children's hair as well.

NOTES

- SECTION III -
RELAXED HAIR

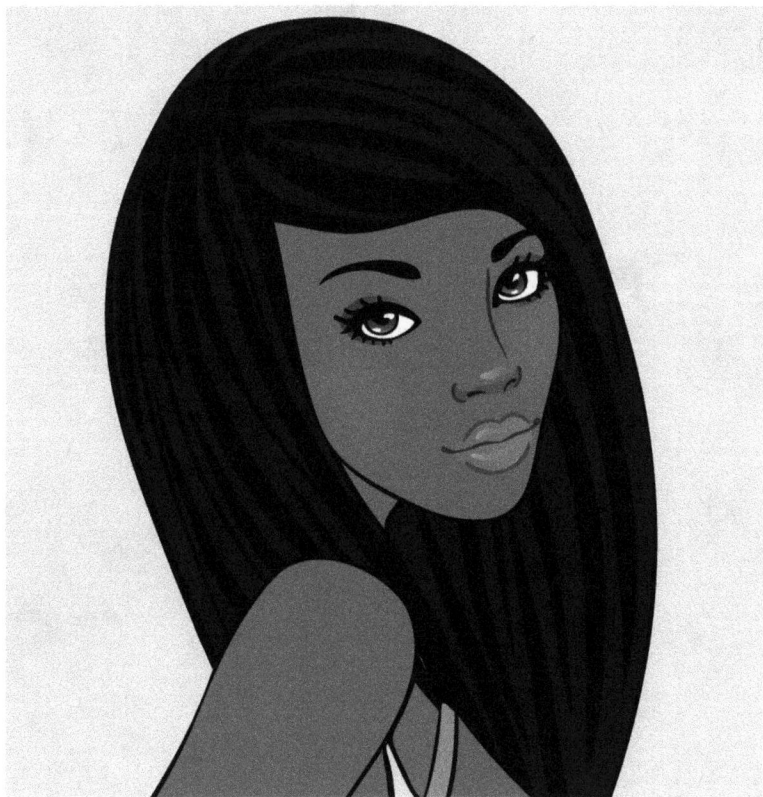

WHAT IS A RELAXER?

Before I begin telling you how to maintain and care for relaxed hair I believe it's important that you know exactly what a relaxer is and the process that your hair goes through during the application.

A relaxer is a chemical made of Sodium Hydroxide which is the strongest type of chemical used in some relaxers because it provides the most long lasting and dramatic effects. Sodium Hydroxide is what is used in products that are referred to as "lye" relaxers. There are also relaxers made of Guanidine Hydroxide which is generally referred to as "no-lye" relaxers. However please do not assume that "no-lye" relaxers aren't as strong as "lye" relaxers or potentially less damaging to the hair. The differences between lye and no-lye relaxer formulas result from the chemical compounds responsible for the straightening action. For lye relaxers, this compound is sodium hydroxide. In no-lye relaxers, this compound can either be guanidine, lithium, or potassium hydroxide. Though, no-lye relaxers claim to have no traces of lye (or "caustic soda"), this statement is not entirely true as the guanidine, lithium, and potassium hydroxides are in the same metal hydroxide family as sodium hydroxide. Lye relaxers have naturally higher pHs than no-lye relaxers, and this is the reason why these stronger formulas are generally only available to professional stylists. Regardless of which relaxer you choose the hair and scalp should be in top condition before performing this service.

HOW DOES A RELAXER WORK?

Both lye and "no lye" relaxers are very strong chemicals that work in the same manner by changing the basic structure of the hair shaft. The chemical penetrates the cortex and loosens the natural curl pattern. This inner layer of the hair shaft is not only what gives curly hair its shape but provides strength and elasticity. Once this process is performed it is irreversible. This process produces the effect of straight hair but at the same time leaves hair weak and extremely susceptible to breaking and further damage. Because relaxers strip hair that is naturally dry it is very important to regularly obtain conditioning treatments before and after the service. Relaxers should never be applied to already damaged hair, or on someone who has had scalp damage.

As a general rule the relaxing process should only be used to soften and smooth the curl pattern no more than 80 percent straight. Always leave some room for elasticity – meaning with a slight wave pattern in the hair and room for the thermal heat process to smooth the hair if it is worn straight. Relaxing your hair until its "bone straight" will result in future breakage and damage; leaving in at least 20% of its natural elasticity allows for stronger hair.

One of the major causes for hair loss and damage for relaxed hair wearers is over processed hair. This is why it's strongly recommended that a relaxer is applied only under the direction of a hair care professional with a record of success with healthy hair care and chemical straightening. Over processing which is the excessive use of relaxers on the hair or applying the chemical to already processed or relaxed hair is the most typical misuse of these chemicals. Once the initial relaxer is applied to virgin or natural hair, touch-ups should only be applied to new growth between 6-8 week periods (or more). This however, depends on the rate of hair growth and condition of the hair as advised by your hair care professional. I personally recommend stretching your relaxers out to a minimum of 12 weeks with proper conditioning and protective styling this will allow your hair to rest from the chemicals and provide a stronger distinction line between the new growth and hair that has already been processed to prevent over processing.

Over processing can also occur when applying hair color. It is standard to wait at least 2-4 weeks before applying hair color chemical (or dye) to recently relaxed hair however as a stylist who is more hair care focused I recommend that you make a choice between the two chemical processes never both. Therefore if you want to color your hair it should remain natural OR relax your hair and opt for no peroxide, no ammonia color products which limits your coloring options but is safer for the hair.   Remember the more chemicals applied to hair the greater the possibility of damage may be experienced.

Age should also be considered before applying relaxers. Although your daughters may want to have the hairstyles they see on adults or other young people it is not in a child's best interest to have such harsh chemicals applied to young hair and has the potential to cause damage that could last a lifetime if misused. If your child insists on having straight hair there are other options, blow drying and pressing with a flat iron is the very best option or even setting the hair with magnetic rollers and blowing straight with a blow dryer. Both methods can be done professionally or at home if you have the skill set and will save your child years of trauma.

Relaxed Hair Care

The steps to take to maintain healthy relaxed hair and achieve great lengths are very similar to those listed in the natural hair section. With moisture and deep conditioning being your main priority however there are some additional steps listed below to help keep the relaxed hair structure strong:

1. Eating Habits - Drinking plenty of water and eating healthy foods will always be a major factor in having healthy hair. If you are not a big vegetable eater taking a daily multi vitamin is a great way to provide vitamin supplements to the body.

2. Application – Relaxers both virgin applications and touch ups should always be done by a professional that has a proven track record of relaxed hair maintenance. Just because someone is licensed does not always mean they are good at what they do, do your research, get a consultation and ask questions to test their knowledge. Once you have found someone you are comfortable with I recommend you see them even if it's just for the application. When you try to apply the relaxer yourself or have someone with no knowledge of the chemical perform this service you are at risk of over processing and severely damaging your hair. (Tip – after the relaxer application it is necessary to neutralize the hair to bring it back to its normal Ph.)

3. Stretching - It's recommended that you have a retouch done every 6 – 8 weeks. This is the standard wait time

between relaxer touch ups however I believe 12 weeks should be the minimum. This leads into the next step…

4. Moisturizing – Moisturizing is a very important step in caring for relaxed hair again water is the best moisturizer and increasing your co washing frequency is the best way to receive maximum moisture. If you decide to stretch your relaxers out to 12 weeks moisturizing will prevent a lot of the shedding and breakage that occurs. Moisturizing every 3 – 4 days would be ideal but if that time span is not feasible weekly is the preferred time length to go without washing your hair. Throughout the week you should use a water based moisturizer like Luster's Pink Oil Moisturizer daily on your ends to prevent dry and split ends. Avoid putting the crème on your hair shaft or at the scalp so that it won't weigh the hair down and to maintain body.

5. Deep Conditioning – As a result of stretching out your relaxer over a 12 week period it is imperative that you deep condition weekly with a moisturizing deep conditioner of your choice. This eliminates the shedding and breakage that usually occurs during the wait period.

6. Treatment – A protein treatment every 6 weeks is mandatory! Because your hair strands are completely

broken down and stripped of oils and proteins it is very important that your regimen includes replacing the elements that you have taken out. Protein treatments keep the hair strong and eliminates shedding and breaking. Aphogee has a great heavy protein treatment that can only be used every 6 weeks but there are also light protein treatments that I will list in the products list that can be used on a weekly basis.

7. Heat Styling – With relaxed hair we tend to use curling irons and flat irons more frequently to maintain a sleek look however this is one of the major culprits of dry, brittle and damaged hair. Heat appliances should not be applied to the hair more than once a week if done properly. With the proper tools and products a thermal straightening or blow dry should last you until your next wash (no longer than a week). A great alternative to curling irons are flexi rods or pin curling the hair to form curls. If you are doing your hair at home investing in professional grade appliances and learning how to properly use these tools will save your hair a great deal. Check out www.undiscovereddiva.com in the tips and gratuities section for blow drying tips and details on the difference between flat irons and blow dryers on the market.

8. Length Retention – Last but not least protective styling is the best way to retain length. Wearing buns, twists, chignons or any style that keeps your fragile ends from rubbing against clothes and weather elements prevents split and breaking ends giving you the opportunity to achieve great lengths.

Quick Tip - If you opt to relax at home please note there are customary neutralizers included in your relaxer kits however it is also a good idea to complete the neutralization process with an Apple Cider Vinegar rinse. A rinse of 1/4 cup apple cider vinegar diluted in 1 to 1 1/2 cups water is also a great and safe way to neutralize the alkalinity of a relaxer while tightly closing the cuticle which leaves the hair with a natural shine.

PRODUCT RECOMMENDATIONS

When it comes to products to use for relaxed hair it's a good idea to invest in higher quality products because of the transformation that occurs during the relaxing process. I've listed some products that worked great for many of my relaxed clients.

Crème Moisturizers – used for daily moisturizing. Apply a dime sized amount to the ends before setting on flexi rods, wrapping or pin curling at night and cover with a satin scarf or bonnet.

- Luster's Pink Oil Moisturizer
- Mizani Rose H2O Conditioning Hairdress
- Mizani H2O Intense Nighttime Treatment

Shampoos and Conditioners – Although I highly recommend that shampooing is done once a month if you have to get some lather using no sulfate no parabens shampoos are the better option because they contain less surfactants and remember one shampoo does the trick.

- Aveda Dry Remedy Shampoo and Conditioner
- Giovanni Brand Shampoo and Conditioners
- Shea Moisture Brand Shampoos and Conditioners

Deep Conditioning Treatments – These treatments should be used on a weekly basis preferably with heat by sitting under a dryer for 15 min or a wrapped towel and let penetrate for 45 min. Whether natural or relaxed I recommend mixing olive oil the deep conditioners to combat dryness and give shine.

- Aveda Dry Remedy Moisture Masque
- Kerastase Brand Deep Treatments
- Keracare Treatments and Masques

Protein Treatments – Providing protein to the hair is a step that should not be missed for anyone who has relaxed hair. There are two ways to add protein to the hair you can do a heavy protein treatment every 6 – 8 weeks or a weekly light protein treatment. Some people complain that using the heavy treatments leave their hair hard and brittle. If you have had that experience remember to always follow the manufacturer's instructions or at minimum try a light protein treatment to add some of the element back into your hair shaft.

- Aphogee Two Step Protein Treatment is a heavy protein treatment and should be used every 6-8 weeks.
- Aphogee Keratin 2 Minute Reconstructor is a follicle building treatment for damaged, dry, brittle hair that can be used weekly.
- Aveda Damage Remedy Shampoo and Conditioner contain protein from the quinoa seed and are light enough to be used weekly.
- Aveda Damage Remedy Intensive Restructuring Treatment can also be used as a weekly deep treatment.

There are a variety of protein treatments and reconstructors on the market but the three named above are what have worked for me in the past.

Any hair that has been chemically processed is at its weakest state but that does not mean that you cannot have healthy hair.

Whether you wear your hair short and chic or long and luxurious be sure to take extra special care of your relaxed strands by moisturizing, deep conditioning and rebuilding the shaft by adding protein.

Quick Tip - Instead *of getting your relaxer every 6-8 weeks get a protein treatment and stretch out your relaxer service to 12 weeks reducing your chemical service to 4 times a year instead of the recommended 6.*

NOTES

- SECTION IV -
Color Treated Hair

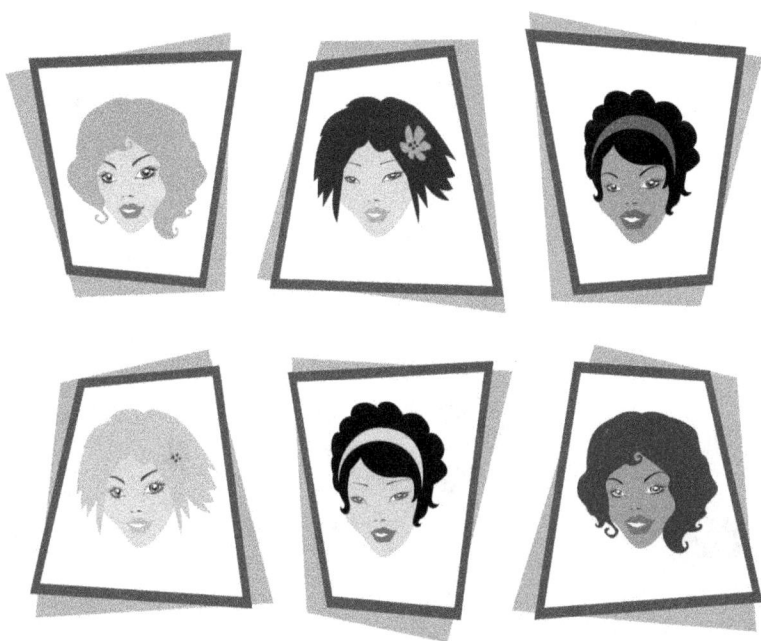

Color Treated Hair

Taking the steps to maintain proper moisture and protein balances within the hair shaft is important especially if you have color-treated your hair with anything other than a color rinse. Rinses and temporary colors sit on top of the hair shaft which is why they wash away after a few shampoos. However semi permanent and permanent color procedures penetrate into the hair shaft leaving the hair more porous and dryer than untreated hair.

It's always best to use moisturizing shampoos and conditioners specifically made for color-treated hair to help prolong the vibrancy of your color. Using regular shampoos can cause your color to appear dull quickly and as mentioned before shampooing can dry your hair out even more which causes breakage in the long run. When washing your hair keep your water in the warm to cool range to avoid stripping the color and remember to protect your hair while swimming in chlorinated pools. Below are a few products you will need to ensure you have the healthiest, color-treated hair:

- L'ANZA Swim and Sun Hair Care Products – this line is specifically designed for protection from chlorinated pools and the UVA/B rays of the sun. The chelating shampoo removes chlorine and minerals that cause the hair to become dry and lack color and shine.

- Moisturizing Shampoo specifically for color treated hair. L'ANZA also makes a line of shampoos and conditioners for color treated hair however there are many others on the market that work just as well.

- Moisturizing Deep Conditioner – refer to recommendations in the relaxed or natural hair section. (Products listed below)
    o Aveda Dry Remedy Moisture Masque
    o Kerastase Brand Deep Treatments
    o Keracare Treatments and Masques

- Protein/Reconstructor Conditioner - refer to recommendations in the relaxed or natural hair section. (Products listed below)
    o Aphogee Two Step Protein Treatment is a heavy protein treatment and should be used every 6-8 weeks.

o Aphogee Keratin 2 Minute Reconstructor is a
   follicle building treatment for damaged, dry,
   brittle hair that can be used weekly.

o Aveda Damage Remedy Shampoo and
   Conditioner contain protein from the quinoa
   seed and are light enough to be used weekly.

o Aveda Damage Remedy Intensive Restructuring
   Treatment can also be used as a weekly deep
   treatment.

You will notice that I made a point of indicating each product should be moisturizing and that's because color treated hair needs more moisture and upkeep than untreated hair. Following each wash with a moisturizing conditioner for at least 20-30 minutes will aid tremendously in preventing the hair from becoming dry and brittle. It's recommended that you forgo any heat styling for at least the first 2 weeks following a color process. Hot oil treatments or apple cider vinegar rinses are also options. They do well in keeping the cuticle smooth and soft.

To keep your colors looking fresh after using permanent or semi-permanent color, consider getting a glaze or color rinse in between salon visits. Color rinses help maintain the correct tone of color and help lessen the chemical damage to the hair shaft.

Keeping your color-treated hair in optimal condition may take a little more time and attention. But as long as you are giving your hair both the needed protein and moisturizing components it needs, your color treated hair will grow healthily!

NOTES

- SECTION V –
HAIR ENHANCEMENTS
& HAIR LOSS

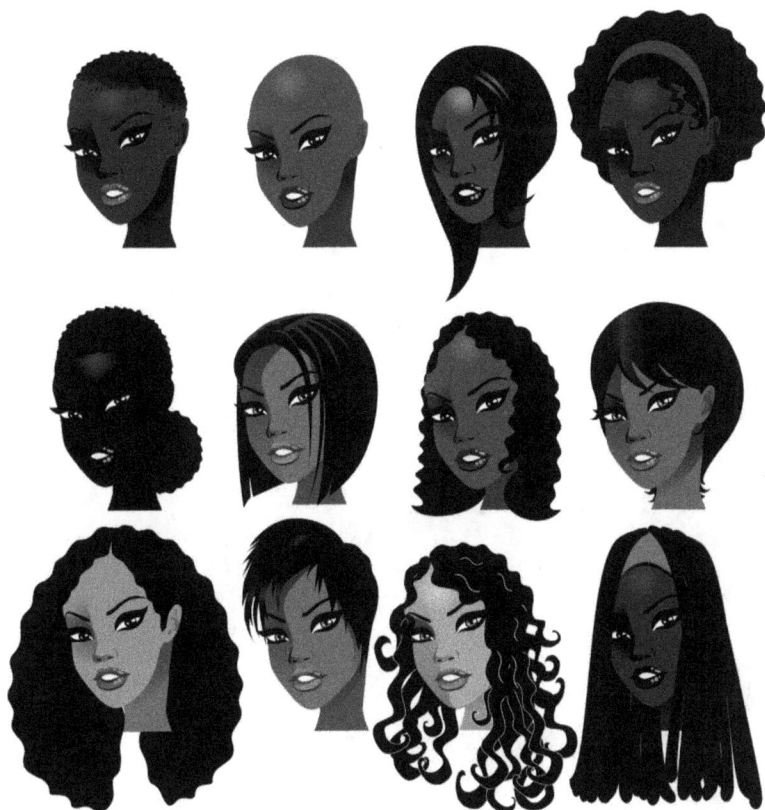

Scalp Disorders

Weaves, braids, twists and wigs are great protective styles and provide options for a new look but they can also be very damaging if not done properly. The use of thermal or chemical hair straightening, and hair braiding or weaving are examples of styling techniques that place African American women at high risk for various "traumatic" alopecia's. Under normal circumstances we lose hair everyday as it's a process in the hairs growth cycle. However over 63 million people in the United States suffer from abnormal hair loss. Although it may not be recognized by the medical community it's evident that hair loss has an emotional impact and cause anguish to the sufferer. Results from a study that investigated perceptions of bald and balding men showed that compared to men who had hair bald men were perceived as:

- Less physically attractive
- Less assertive
- Less successful
- Less personally likable

On the other hand, for women, abnormal hair loss is particularly devastating. Women tend to have a greater emotional investment in their appearance and abnormal hair loss can be very traumatic. The majority of women who suffer from hair loss feel anxious, helpless and less attractive and for African American women they resort to wearing hair extensions in the form of braids and weaves to assist in growth but many times these options only make the problem worse.

There are many types of alopecia's including androgenic alopecia, alopecia areata and post partum alopecia but one of the most common side effects seen on women who wear braids and weaves is traction alopecia.

Traction alopecia is a hair loss condition caused by damage to the dermal papilla and hair follicle by constant pulling or tension over a long period of time. It often occurs to people who wears tight braids, especially "cornrows" that lead to high tension, pulling and breakage of hair. Now imagine having your hair in tight cornrows and the tension from sewing tracks of weave over those braids! Just the thought gives me a headache but before I explain how to alleviate this issue I will give you more information on this condition.

Traction alopecia is reversible if diagnosed early, but may lead to permanent hair loss if it is undetected over a period of time.

Hair loss is often in the frontal and temporal regions, but also depends on the hair style. Those who wear cornrows, the area most commonly affected is that adjacent to the region that is braided.

Traction Alopecia can also occur as a result of over processing of the hair. Chemical treatment of hair with dyes, bleaches, or straighteners disrupts the keratin structure in a manner that reduces its strength making the hair fragile and causing heavy fall out to occur with brushing or combing.

PREVENTING ALOPECIA

The key to stopping traction alopecia is detecting it early. Hair styles that put unnecessary strain on the hair root must be changed for looser, gentler hair styles. Women who suspect they may be vulnerable to traction alopecia should take action immediately to change their hair style or treatment methods and by all means, take the time to see a dermatologist. Unfortunately, no medical treatment is available to reverse late-stage traction alopecia. Hair grafts have been identified as the only practical solution.

Now I don't mean to scare you away from wearing or trying weaves or even braided hairstyles because there are ways to get these styles without the risk of getting traction alopecia. Below you will find a list of weaving and braiding style methods that allows women to continue to wear their enhancements worry free.

WEAVE AND WIG MAINTENANCE

There are many ways to install a weave, they can be bonded, sewn or fused to the hair however wearing a wig is the best alternative to any form of weaving because it allows you to remove the hair piece daily and care for your hair underneath. Always remember to wear a wig cp underneath to protect your hair and steer clear of bonding lace front wigs to your hair line. If you opt to wear a lace front wig it is best to wear it as a full cap wig instead of gluing the hair to your hairline. Lace front wigs were intentionally made for women who suffer from baldness for medical related issues however they have gotten the attention of the regular consumer and many women are damaging their hairlines to achieve a "realistic look" with the lace front wig. If you are blessed to have hair don't ruin it stick to half wigs or full cap wigs so that you will not have to really need a lace front later down the road.

Bonded Weave

Bonded Weave also known as glued in weave gives the quickest and flattest results. A special weave glue is used to attach individual tracks to areas where you may want more length or a hint of color. When adding weave using the bonding method be sure to attach the track to the base of your hair root getting as close to the scalp as possible. Many feel this is the unhealthiest option for your hair but if it's removed properly and worn for no longer than a week you hair will not suffer any major damage. When removing bonded weave the trick is to be sure to oil the area with oil sheen or even olive oil where the track rests on your hair to ensure maximum slip; that why it will not tug any hairs. Also a common mistake many women make is trying to re-glue a bonded track. When the track begins to give way it's in your best interest to oil and remove the remaining hair from your scalp. Constantly rebonding the weave results in hair breakage and thinning.

Sew In Method

Sewing in weaves can be both the safest and the worst way to install hair extensions. A good install can last a client up to three months and allow your hair a rest between chemical services and manipulation while a bad install can cause traction alopecia as described above. To avoid the worst case scenario when getting a full head a weave a stylist that's hair care focused would never suggest enclosing your entire head of hair. For your hairs sake it is always a best practice to leave the weakest and most fragile sections out not only so that the install can look as real as possible but to also avoid damage. Leaving out the perimeter of your hair line and nape as well as a horseshoe section in the crown is the first step of avoiding traction alopecia. Also your stylist should also NEVER braid the foundation of your weave extremely tight. If you find yourself wincing while he/she is braiding ask that they loosen up the braids or schedule an appointment with someone who knows better. Do not let anyone convince you it's supposed to be extremely tight in order to get better results you will save yourself and your hair a lot of grief.

Weave Maintenance

When it comes to maintaining your hair under a sew in weave it's very important that you cleanse your scalp regularly. Using a dry shampoo or a product like Sea breeze Astringent to cleanse the scalp is the best way to product buildup and allows your scalp to breathe. You may also wash your hair the traditional way however after washing your hair, be sure to sit under a hooded dryer until your hair and the foundation is completely dry. Leaving weaves damp can cause mildew and fungus that will also damage and make it a tangled mess when it's time for removal.

BRAIDS AND TWISTS

Other popular styles among African American women are box braids, kinky twists, Senegalese twists and cornrows. These styles are also attributed to the rise in traction alopecia but there are ways to still wear them without suffering such devastating consequences.

The first step would be to use quality human hair when getting braids and twists. Human hair now comes in all textures from straight to kinky and everything in between. It may carry a hefty price tag but when it comes to the health of your hair it's definitely worth the investment and the hair can be washed and reused. If the prices just aren't in your budget at the moment synthetic hair can be used however just as you would with natural hair to prevent damage you should keep the hair moist as often as possible by spraying it once in the morning and once at night with a concoction of water and conditioner. This keeps the hair soft and does not allow the synthetic hair to dry your hair out and strip it of its natural oils. Keeping synthetic hair moist also prevents it from causing split ends. Think of synthetic hair as barbed wire, as your hair grows the manmade fibers cut through your hair leaving it damaged and usually having to get trimmed upon removal.

The second step is to avoid going to a braider or stylist that insists on braiding your hair extremely tight. Beauty should not hurt! If your head hurts, it's because your hair is braided too tightly, or you have too much extension hair added. A braider may braid tightly so that the style lasts as long as possible but tight tension is not good for your hair, hairline and scalp. Again this practice is what results in traction alopecia and it is not worth a hairstyle to last a week more. Medium tension is best for any type of braided style it may not last as long as tight braids, but your hairline will not thin or disappear as a result.

If you're a victim of headache-inducing braids you should immediately remove the braids. Friends and stylists may recommend that you wet the braids, take an aspirin but these practices will not save the fragile hair being torn from your scalp! Once removed vow to never go to that stylist again and give your hair a rest from the tension; treat your hair using the relaxed or natural hair care tips listed above and try to find a professional hair braider that is also a hair care specialist.

EPILOGUE

Does Beauty = Self Esteem?

Everyone has had bad hair days and studies have shown that these "bad hair days" affect individuals self esteem increasing self doubt, social insecurities and becoming more self critical. According to "The Psychological, Interpersonal and Social Effects of Bad Hair" women tend to feel more disgraced, embarrassed, ashamed or self consciousness when they believe their physical appearance is not up to par. This leads one to find more character flaws that go beyond their appearance affecting their confidence. These strong emotions of beauty and self esteem is due largely to media portrayal of what is considered ideal beauty and while it affects people of all races and nationalities I believe the African American community is affected the most. However your own sense of self worth should never rely on whether you think your hair is beautiful or not. To be quite honest it's really the other way around meaning your beauty increases when you add self esteem. Beauty alone will not give you the confidence you seek; true beauty comes from the process of building real self esteem. Self esteem does not rely on what other people may think of you and the first step to gaining self esteem includes self realization, self knowledge, self awareness and self respect. Spend some time discovering your own inner qualities and appreciating them. Express these qualities freely for the benefit of others and you will gradually come to know your own unique true beauty whether your hair is long, short, straight, kinky, curly, wavy!

FAQ'S

Q: How do I decide what shampoo and conditioner to use?

A: The most important thing that a shampoo and conditioner for African American hair should do is provide moisture. If your hair needs specific treatments you can always add those later on but there has to be a good foundation first. It might be a while before you find your perfect match or you might get lucky and find something you like right away. Just remember sulfate and parabens free are always your best options and never buy a shampoo because of how it smells, but for what it does to your hair.

Q: How do I stop my hair from breaking?

A: There's a lot you can do to counteract breakage problems with your hair. First start with drinking more water dehydrated hair is usually the culprit. Once you increase your water intake both internally and by psychically moisturizing by increasing your wash frequency to at least once a week I would suggest the following:

- If you wear your hair relaxed stretch out your touch ups to 12 weeks and replace your touch ups with heavy protein treatments.

- Use your flat iron or curling iron less frequently and opt for flexi rods or pin curls to set the hair.
- Invest in a satin pillow case and be sure to protect your hair with a satin bonnet or scarf.
- Wear more protective styles keeping your fragile ends from rubbing against your clothes and causing breakage.

Q. How often should I wash my hair?
A. Every three days if possible however if your lifestyle and schedule does not permit then once a week is the absolute longest length of time between washing. Also it's a good idea to co wash or use no sulfate shampoos to prevent drying and damaging your hair.

Q. I color treat my hair every six weeks. I've been told that shampooing my hair everyday fades my hair faster. What do you recommend to keep my color from fading?
A. A cream based cleansing cream is the best product to use for color treated hair to avoid stripping the color or any shampoo and conditioner line that's specifically formulated for color treated hair. L'Anza is a good line to try.

Q. I've been relaxing my hair for years how do I go natural?

A. Transitioning from a relaxed to natural style is not as overwhelming as you may think. Simply stop relaxing it. Here are a couple of ways to go about it.

- You can opt for rod sets and twist outs or continue to heat style without worrying about the damaging effects of your relaxed hair.

- You can cut it and start over. Note - Cutting your hair can be a very emotional experience. But I've found many women find it liberating.

- If you're not ready to take the plunge and cut your hair off, you can wear weaves or hair extensions. Weaves are a great way to transition through the process.

ABOUT THE AUTHOR

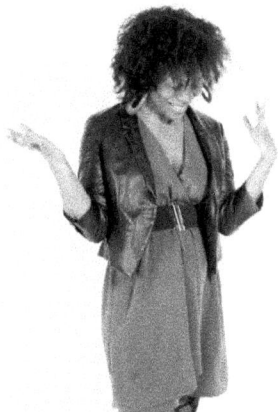

Who is Terrie Lauren?

Author, Blogger, Stylist and Entrepreneur, Terrie Lauren was born and raised in Brooklyn, NY.

Although she always had a passion for fashion and beauty, which was evident in her youth through constant experimentations on her own hair with cuts and colors and unique style; Terrie decided to take the more traditional career route by completing college and entering the corporate world.

After years of not feeling like she fit in with the suits and being bored with every job she had she decided to take a leap of faith and pursue her passion by attending Aveda beauty school in New York City. Upon entering the program she realized this was her "call of duty" and has been loyal to the craft ever since!

Her passion for hair has lead her to managing salons, working on photo shoots and on the sets of major TV networks. With a love for highly textured and curly hair Terrie decided to share her knowledge of healthy hair care with the world in her debut book titled "Undiscovered Diva – Reclaim your Natural Beauty".

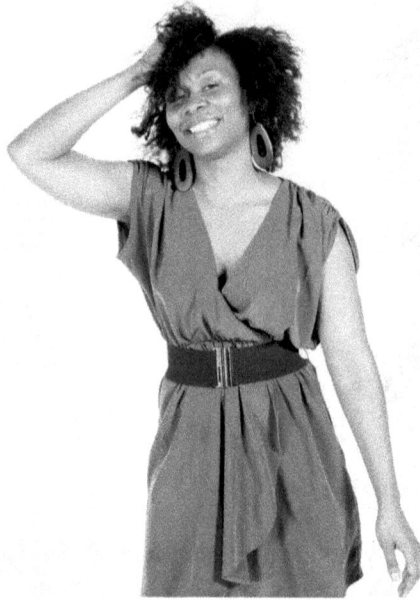

You can visit Terrie online at
WWW.UNDISCOVEREDDIVA.COM
WHERE SHE BLOGS ABOUT HER
CAREER JOURNEY AND PROVIDES
HAIR AND PRODUCT TIPS.

To book Terrie for your
WORKSHOP, SEMINAR OR
CONFERENCE PLEASE EMAIL
INFO@UNDISCOVEREDDIVA.COM